SJOGREN'S SYNDROME DIET COOKBOOK

Delicious Recipes For Managing Dry Mouth, Eyes, Fatigue, And Autoimmune Symptoms With Nutrient-Rich, Anti-Inflammatory Meals, And Guidelines – All You Need To Know

DR. AMARI VALERIE

TABLE OF CONTENTS

BONUS:

7 days meal plan recipes, ingredients, and detailed preparatory guidelines for Sjogren's Syndrome

7 Desserts procedural recipes for Sjogren's Syndrome and guidelines

7 Smoothies procedural recipes for Sjogren's Syndrome and guidelines

DISCLAIMER

The information provided in this book, is for educational and informational purposes only and is not intended as medical advice. The content is not a substitute for professional medical advice, diagnosis, or treatment. Always seek the advice of your physician or other qualified health provider with any questions you may have regarding a medical condition. Never disregard professional medical advice or delay in seeking it because of something you have read in this book.

The dietary suggestions and recipes in this book are based on general guidelines and may not be suitable for everyone. Individual responses to foods can vary, and it is important to consult with a healthcare professional before making any significant changes to your diet.

The author and publisher of this book do not claim to cure or treat any medical condition. The information provided is based on research and personal experience and is intended to help readers make informed decisions about their diet and health.

Furthermore, I the author do not endorse any specific products, brands, treatments, or services that may be mentioned in this book. Any references to products, services, websites, or organizations are provided for informational purposes only and do not constitute an endorsement or recommendation by the author. The inclusion of such references does not imply any association, sponsorship, or affiliation between the author and the referenced entities.

The recipes and dietary suggestions in this book are designed to be safe and healthful. However, readers should use their own discretion and consult with a healthcare professional when necessary, especially if they have allergies, sensitivities, or other dietary restrictions.

By using this book, you acknowledge and agree that the author and publisher shall not be held liable for any loss or damage, including but not limited to special, incidental, consequential, or other damages, resulting from the use of the information and recipes contained in this book.

ABOUT THIS BOOK

This "Sjogren's Syndrome Diet Cookbook" is a comprehensive resource for individuals who are attempting to navigate the intricacies of living with Sjogren's Syndrome. The definition, symptoms, causes, and risk factors of the condition are all detailed in the introductory sections, which also explore the diagnostic process and prevalent complications. This provides a fundamental understanding of the condition. This foundational work underscores the critical role that diet plays in the management of Sjogren's Syndrome symptoms, emphasizing the significance of nutrition in the mitigation of the effects of this autoimmune disorder.

This cookbook then transitions to an examination of the impact of diet on autoimmune conditions, with a particular emphasis on inflammation. It assists readers in making well-informed dietary decisions by highlighting the advantages of anti-inflammatory and nutrient-dense foods. The significance of hydration in the management of Sjogren's Syndrome symptoms is a recurring theme. It offers a clear roadmap for dietary adjustments by providing practical advice on which foods to avoid preventing exacerbating symptoms.

The meticulous coverage of nutrient-rich ingredients underscores the importance of essential vitamins and minerals for individuals with Sjogren's Syndrome. The compendium advocates for the advantages of whole foods over processed alternatives, as well as antioxidants and nutrients. Practical meal planning advice is offered to guarantee that readers can effortlessly integrate these nutrient-dense ingredients into their daily routines.

This cookbook contains cooking techniques that are specifically designed to alleviate symptoms. It provides methods for managing a parched mouth, ensuring that food remains hydrated and palatable, and facilitating the swallowing of meals. Additionally, this book addresses the importance of utilizing time-saving culinary techniques and adapting recipes to optimize nutrient density, thereby ensuring that meal preparation is feasible despite the fatigue and discomfort that are frequently associated with Sjogren's Syndrome.

Frequently asked questions (FAQs) and common concerns pertain to practical matters, including managing weight, modifying recipes for dietary restrictions, dining out, and managing fatigue and tired eyes during meal preparation.

These sections offer practical solutions and modifications to assist readers in maintaining a balanced diet without overtaxing their already overtaxed systems.

This cookbook encompasses a diverse selection of meal types, including energy-boosting breakfasts, sustaining lunches, health-focused dinners, and gratifying nibbles and deserts, as it progresses through specific chapters. Each composition is tailored to the specific requirements of Sjogren's Syndrome patients, with a focus on hydration, anti-inflammatory ingredients, and simplicity of preparation.

Breakfasts emphasize hydration and energy, while lunches and dinners emphasize sustained energy and optimal health by incorporating protein-rich main dishes, salads, and substantial stews. Snacks and desserts provide individuals with Sjogren's

Syndrome with fast, nutritious alternatives that accommodate their dietary restrictions and appetites.

The suggestions for meal planning and preparation are comprehensively described, including weekly strategies, batch culinary techniques, and a grocery purchasing guide. A 7-day meal plan, which includes detailed recipes and preparatory guidelines, is included in this cookbook to ensure that readers can seamlessly incorporate these recommendations into their routines. Procedural recipes for smoothies and desserts provide a greater degree of enjoyment and variety.

This cookbook concludes by providing lifestyle recommendations for the management of Sjogren's Syndrome. It underscores the significance of maintaining normal sleep, managing stress, maintaining hydration, and engaging in regular exercise. Additionally, readers are provided with opportunities for further assistance and solidarity through the promotion of community resources and support. This "Sjogren's Syndrome Diet Cookbook" is not merely a compilation of recipes; it is a valuable resource for the comprehensive management of lifestyle. This is the result of the holistic approach.

CHAPTER ONE

Introduction

Greetings and thank you for visiting the Sjogren's Syndrome Diet Cookbook! Sjogren's syndrome is a chronic autoimmune disorder that primarily affects the moisture-producing glands in the body, including the salivary and mucus glands. This guide is intended to assist you in managing the dietary aspects of the condition. Symptoms can be alleviated and your overall quality of life can be enhanced by implementing straightforward yet effective dietary modifications.

Comprehending Sjogren's Syndrome

Sjogren's syndrome is an autoimmune disorder in which the body's immune system inadvertently targets its moisture-producing organs, resulting in dryness in the pharynx, eyes, and other regions. parched eyes, parched saliva, fatigue, joint pain, and difficulty swallowing are among the symptoms. It is essential to comprehend the nature of this condition to effectively manage its symptoms and complications.

Significance Of Diet In Symptom Management

The symptoms of Sjogren's syndrome are significantly influenced by diet. Dryness and inflammation can be exacerbated by certain foods, while others can alleviate discomfort and improve overall health.

By making well-informed dietary decisions, you can enhance your quality of life and more effectively manage your symptoms. For instance, the body can experience a reduction in inflammation and dehydration by consuming foods that are high in omega-3 fatty acids, such as flaxseeds and salmon.

Risk Factors And Causes

Sjogren's syndrome is believed to be caused by a combination of genetic, environmental, and hormonal factors, although the precise cause remains uncertain. Sjogren's syndrome develops more frequently in women than in men, and it frequently co-occurs with other autoimmune conditions, such as lupus or rheumatoid arthritis. Individuals can take proactive measures to manage their condition and mitigate its impact on their daily lives by comprehending the potential causes and risk factors.

Common Complications And The Diagnosis Process

The diagnosis of Sjogren's syndrome can be difficult due to the diversity of its symptoms, which can be akin to those of other conditions. Specialized tests, including salivary gland biopsies and blood testing, are frequently required to make an accurate diagnosis, in addition to a comprehensive medical history and physical examination. Furthermore, Sjogren's syndrome may result in complications, including an elevated risk of lymphoma, oral yeast infections, and dental decay. To mitigate these complications and preserve overall health, it is imperative to implement proactive management and consistent monitoring.

The Impact Of Diet On Autoimmune Conditions

A diet that is specifically designed to manage autoimmune conditions such as Sjogren's syndrome can be instrumental in the reduction of symptoms and the enhancement of overall health. Individuals can effectively manage their symptoms and promote wellness by emphasizing nutrient-rich foods that support the immune system and reduce inflammation.

The Impact of Diet on Inflammation: Specific nutrients can either promote or combat inflammation in the body. Individuals with Sjogren's syndrome need to prioritize anti-inflammatory nutrients to alleviate the pain and distress that are associated with inflammation.

The consumption of foods such as oily salmon that are high in omega-3 fatty acids, leafy greens that are abundant in antioxidants, and turmeric, which has anti-inflammatory properties, can assist in the management of inflammation.

Nutrient-Dense Foods and Their Advantages: The consumption of nutrient-dense foods is essential for the maintenance of overall health and the management of symptoms of Sjogren's syndrome, as it provides essential vitamins, minerals, and antioxidants.

Colorful fruits and vegetables, whole cereals, lean proteins such as poultry and legumes, and healthy fats from sources such as avocados and almonds can provide a diverse array of nutrients to support immune function and overall well-being.

Anti-Inflammatory Foods: The inclusion of a diverse array of anti-inflammatory foods in one's diet can serve to mitigate symptoms associated with Sjogren's syndrome. By incorporating foods such as ginger, which is renowned for its anti-inflammatory properties, and green tea, which contains polyphenols, inflammation can be reduced, and symptoms such as fatigue and joint pain can be alleviated.

Foods to Avoid: Certain foods can exacerbate inflammation and exacerbate the symptoms of Sjogren's syndrome.

It is crucial to restrict or avoid processed foods that are high in refined carbohydrates and unhealthy lipids, as well as foods that contain gluten and dairy, as they may induce inflammation in certain individuals. Furthermore, it is recommended that individuals with Sjogren's syndrome refrain from consuming caffeine and alcohol, as they can exacerbate dehydration and dehydrate the body.

Hydration is essential for individuals with Sjogren's syndrome to manage dehydration, particularly in the pharynx and eyes.

To mitigate the distress associated with dryness and maintain moisture levels in the body, it is important to consume an adequate quantity of water throughout the day and incorporate hydrating foods such as cucumbers, watermelons, and soups.

CHAPTER TWO

Ingredients That Are Abundant In Nutrients

When developing a diet that is beneficial for Sjogren's Syndrome, it is important to prioritize nutrient-rich ingredients such as lean proteins, nuts, seeds, legumes, and leafy vegetables.

It is imperative to manage the symptoms of Sjogren's disease, as these foods are abundant in essential vitamins and minerals that are essential for overall health and immune function. Aim for a balanced diet that meets the body's nutritional requirements by incorporating a diverse selection of vibrant fruits and vegetables.

Essential Vitamins and Minerals: Guarantee that your diet contains essential vitamins and minerals, including calcium, vitamin D, omega-3 fatty acids, and vitamin C. These nutrients are essential for the maintenance of bone health, the reduction of inflammation, and the support of immune function, all of which are particularly critical for those with Sjogren's Syndrome. Incorporate sources of these nutrients into your meals, such as citrus fruits for vitamin C, oily fish like salmon for omega-3s, and leafy vegetables for calcium.

Sjogren's Syndrome Superfoods: The high levels of antioxidants and anti-inflammatory properties in superfoods such as blueberries, spinach, kale, and turmeric are beneficial for individuals with Sjogren's Syndrome.

For instance, blueberries are abundant in antioxidants that aid in the prevention of oxidative stress and the reduction of inflammation. Turmeric, on the other hand, is recognized for its anti-inflammatory properties (Curcumin). These nutrients can be incorporated into your diet to alleviate symptoms and promote overall health.

Processed Foods vs. Whole Foods: To promote your health while managing Sjogren's Syndrome, prioritize whole foods over processed foods. Essential nutrients are supplied by whole foods, including fruits, vegetables, whole cereals, and lean proteins, which are devoid of the added carbohydrates, unhealthy fats, and preservatives that are frequently present in processed foods.

By selecting whole foods, you can more effectively manage your nutrient intake and prevent potential catalysts for inflammation or digestive issues that are associated with processed foods.

Antioxidants are essential for individuals with Sjogren's Syndrome, as they assist in the neutralization of free radicals and the reduction of oxidative stress in the body. To mitigate inflammation and safeguard against cell injury, incorporate antioxidant-rich foods, including almonds, seeds, leafy vegetables, and berries, into your diet. By incorporating a diverse array of antioxidant-rich foods into your diet, you can alleviate symptoms and enhance your overall health.

Meal Planning Tips: When preparing meals for Sjogren's Syndrome, it is important to incorporate a diverse selection of nutrient-rich foods and to take into account any dietary restrictions or sensitivities.

Strive to consume nutritious meals that consist of a variety of fruits and vegetables, whole cereals, lean proteins, and healthy lipids. To ensure that meals remain engaging and pleasurable, experiment with a variety of recipes and culinary methods. Furthermore, considering meal preparation can help you save time and guarantee that you always have nutritious options available, thereby facilitating the maintenance of your dietary objectives and the effective management of your condition.

Cooking Strategies For Symptom Management

It is imperative to take into account the symptoms of Sjogren's Syndrome, including parched mouth and digestive difficulties when cooking. To preserve moisture in your dishes, choose moist culinary methods such as simmering, braising, or stewing.

Incorporate flavorful ingredients such as herbs, seasonings, and citrus to improve the taste of a dish without the need for additional salt or sugar.

Chop or incorporate foods to facilitate chewing and swallowing, and consider incorporating sauces, gravies, or broths to enhance the moistness of meals. Finally, to promote overall health, it is important to prioritize nutrient-dense foods such as verdant greens, lean proteins, and whole grains.

Cooking Strategies For Individuals With Dry Mouth

While cooking, it is necessary to employ deliberate strategies to alleviate a parched mouth. Ensure that you are adequately hydrated by consuming sugar-free chocolates or drinking water throughout the day to increase saliva production.

To prevent dehydration in dishes, employ moist culinary methods such as poaching or baking with additional liquids.

Incorporate hydrating ingredients, such as fruits, vegetables, and yogurt, into recipes to increase the moisture content. Refrain from consuming foods that are excessively fiery or salted, as they can exacerbate dry mouth symptoms. Additionally, consider utilizing a humidifier in the kitchen to ensure that the air is adequately moistened.

Facilitating The Ingestion Of Food

It is imperative to modify meals for individuals who are having difficulty ingesting. Ease of swallowing is achieved by cooking or pureeing foods until they achieve a fluid consistency. To reduce the risk of choking, incorporate delicate textures such as mashed potatoes, cooked vegetables, and tender proteins into dishes.

To facilitate swallowing, cut food into tiny, bite-sized portions and steer clear of tough or fibrous foods that may be difficult to metabolize. To facilitate consumption, experiment with thickening agents such as yogurt or liquefied fruits to improve the texture of soups, sauces, and smoothies.

Preserving The Freshness And Flavor Of Food

Consider a variety of methods to preserve the moisture and flavor of your meals. Before cooking, marinate proteins in fragrant liquids or tenderizing agents to enhance flavor and imbue moisture. To prevent dehydration and enhance the depth of flavor, incorporate sauces, garnishes, or condiments into your dishes.

Incorporate high-moisture ingredients, such as avocados, cucumbers, or tomatoes, into salads or sandwiches to provide a revitalizing boost.

To prevent adhering and improve the mouthfeel of dishes, it is recommended to use cooking oils or lipids. Additionally, a small amount of citrus juice or vinegar can be added to brighten up the dish.

Modifying Recipes To Optimize Nutrient Density

Incorporating nutrient-rich ingredients while accommodating dietary restrictions is the primary objective when modifying recipes for nutrient density. To increase the content of fiber and micronutrients, replace refined grains with whole grains such as quinoa, brown rice, or barley. Substitute processed sugars with natural sweeteners, such as honey, maple syrup, or pureed fruits, to reduce the amount of added sugars and increase the intake of vitamins and minerals.

Enhance the nutritional value of dishes by incorporating additional servings of vegetables or incorporating them into sauces, stews, or casseroles.

Investigate the use of plant-based proteins, such as tofu, tempeh, or legumes, to increase the nutrient density of meals and diversify protein sources.

CHAPTER THREE

Frequently Asked Questions And Common Concerns

Common concerns for individuals with Sjogren's Syndrome include the management of symptoms while maintaining a balanced diet. Questions that are frequently posed may include the following: how to maintain food moisture for easier swallowing, which foods to avoid to prevent flare-ups, and how to remain hydrated.

It is essential to comprehend which constituents are inflammatory and which can alleviate symptoms. For instance, the consumption of omega-3-rich foods such as salmon and chia seeds can aid in the reduction of inflammation, while the avoidance of excessively piquant or acidic foods can prevent discomfort.

Managing Fatigue During The Cooking Process

Planning and preparation can significantly alleviate the exhaustion that individuals with Sjogren's Syndrome experience when cooking. Elect to prepare dishes with minimal effort by using a slow cooker or batch cookery. For example, the daily workload is reduced by preparing a substantial quantity of vegetable stew that can be refrigerated and reheated over the course of the week. Furthermore, energy conservation can be achieved by organizing the kitchen to ensure that frequently used items are readily accessible.

Managing Dry Eyes During Meal Preparation

Meal preparation can be significantly impeded by dry eyes. To prevent irritation from smoke or strong aromas, it is important to take regular pauses to apply lubricating eye drops and ensure that the kitchen is well-ventilated. Additionally, the use of wraparound spectacles can safeguard the eyes from arid air. Furthermore, the utilization of pre-chopped vegetables or a food processor can alleviate eye strain and reduce the time spent slicing.

Dining Out With Sjogren's Syndrome

Eating out can be difficult for individuals with Sjogren's Syndrome; however, it is feasible with proper preparation. Inquire with restaurants in advance about their menu options that accommodate dietary restrictions and moisture requirements. Select dishes that contain broths or condiments that are more easily digestible.

For example, a soup-based dish or grilled fish with a mild marinade can be both palatable and appropriate. Additionally, it is beneficial to bring a small container of olive oil to give moisture to dry dishes.

Modifying Recipes To Comply With Dietary Restrictions

It is imperative to modify recipes to accommodate dietary restrictions to effectively manage Sjogren's Syndrome. Substitute common allergens or irritants with appropriate substitutes. For instance, substitute almond milk for dairy milk or gluten-free flour for wheat flour. Incorporating anti-inflammatory ingredients, such as turmeric or ginger, into recipes can also yield additional health advantages.

Maintain a collection of recipes that are adaptable and can be readily modified to accommodate the ingredients that are tolerated.

The fatigue and dietary restrictions that are associated with Sjogren's Syndrome can make weight management a challenging endeavor. Focus on foods that are low in calories and are nutrient-dense, as they provide energy without providing an excessive amount of calories.

For example, a balanced diet can be achieved by increasing the consumption of vegetables, lean proteins like chicken breast or tofu, and healthy lipids like avocado. Regular, moderate exercise, such as yoga or walking, can be a beneficial addition to dietary efforts and can assist in the effective management of weight.

CHAPTER FOUR

Commencing The Sjogren's Syndrome Diet

Begin your journey with the Sjogren's Syndrome Diet by avoiding common trigger foods, including gluten, dairy, and refined carbohydrates, which can exacerbate inflammation and symptoms. Emphasize the consumption of anti-inflammatory foods, including fresh fruits, vegetables, lean proteins, and healthy lipids.

For instance, begin your day with a smoothie that contains chia seeds, almond milk, berries, and spinach. To facilitate your body's adaptation and to more effectively identify foods that may trigger flare-ups, gradually implement these changes in your diet.

It is imperative to comprehend the extent to which Sjogren's Syndrome symptoms are influenced by diet. Inflammation can be induced by specific substances, resulting in increased fatigue and dehydration. For example, foods that are abundant in omega-3 fatty acids, such as salmon and flaxseeds, can alleviate inflammation. Conversely, processed foods that are high in sugar and trans fats can exacerbate their symptoms.

Keeping a food diary can assist in the identification of patterns between dietary choices and symptom flare-ups, allowing you to make informed alterations to your diet. Additionally, it can assist in tracking what you consume.

Establishing Dietary Objectives For Symptom Management

To effectively manage the symptoms of Sjogren's Syndrome, establish specific, achievable dietary objectives. Begin with straightforward goals, such as consuming eight glasses of water daily to alleviate dehydration or incorporating at least one anti-inflammatory food into each meal.

For instance, strive to include a tablespoon of olive oil or a fistful of hazelnuts in your daily diet. Gradually enhance these objectives by incorporating additional nutrient-dense foods and decreasing the consumption of potential trigger foods. Monitor progress and make adjustments as necessary.

Kitchen Tools And Equipment That Are Essential

Provide your kitchen with indispensable appliances that facilitate the preparation of dishes that are suitable for individuals with Sjogren's syndrome. Purchase a high-quality blender for smoothies and soups, a slow cooker for effortless meal preparation, and non-stick cookware to minimize the necessity for oils and lipids. For instance, utilize a slow cooker to prepare a nutritious vegetable stew that includes sweet potatoes, carrots, and lentils. This dish is also mild on the digestive system. These instruments can assist in the simplification of meal preparation and the facilitation of healthy consumption.

Providing Your Pantry With Ingredients That Are Compatible With Sjogren's Syndrome

Ensure that your larder is stocked with ingredients that are compatible with a diet that is favorable to Sjogren's. For nutritious munchies, maintain a diverse selection of whole cereals, including brown rice and quinoa, legumes like chickpeas and lentils, and a variety of nuts and seeds. Incorporate an abundance of seasonings and herbs, such as ginger and turmeric, which possess anti-inflammatory properties.

For instance, a nutritious dish could be prepared by combining quinoa, chickpeas, diced tomatoes, and spinach, and seasoning it with turmeric and cumin to enhance its flavor and health benefits. Maintaining a well-stocked pantry guarantees that you have the necessary ingredients for a nutritious meal at all times.

Developing A Well-Balanced Meal Plan

To manage the symptoms of Sjogren's Syndrome and satisfy your nutritional requirements, it is necessary to incorporate a diverse array of nutrient-dense foods into a well-balanced meal plan. Arrange your meals to include a variety of fruits and vegetables, whole cereals, and lean proteins. For example, a nutritious lunch could consist of grilled chicken breast, quinoa, and steamed broccoli, all drizzled with olive oil. To sustain energy levels throughout the day, incorporate snacks such as apple slices with almond butter or a small fistful of assorted nuts. Preventing dietary tedium and ensuring a diverse array of nutrients can be achieved by consistently rotating your meal options.

CHAPTER FIVE

Breakfast Recipes For Hydration And Energy

Begin your day with meals that are specifically designed to enhance your vitality and preserve your hydration. Choose a breakfast that is both nutritious and replenishing, such as overnight oats that are prepared with almond milk, chia seeds, and fresh cherries. The milk and fruit in this combination provide slow-releasing carbohydrates for energy and hydration. Additionally, you may incorporate a side of Greek yogurt with a drizzle of honey and a scattering of almonds to enhance the protein and healthy fat content.

Smoothies And Juices For Hydration

Smoothies and beverages are an exceptional source of hydration and nutrient intake. Create a green smoothie by combining spinach, cucumber, a green apple, lemon juice, and coconut water. This beverage is not only hydrating, but it is also abundant in vitamins and minerals. For an additional boost, incorporate a handful of flaxseeds or chia seeds into your smoothie to obtain omega-3 fatty acids, which are effective in reducing inflammation.

Nutritious Breakfast Bowls

Combine a variety of wholesome ingredients in a single meal to create nutritious breakfast dishes. For example, a quinoa breakfast dish can be made by combining cooked quinoa, diced avocado, cherry tomatoes, black beans, and a sprinkling of feta cheese. Drizzle with lemon juice and olive oil to enhance the flavor and provide anti-inflammatory benefits. This bowl is abundant in protein, fiber, and healthy lipids, which will ensure that you remain satisfied and energized for the duration of the morning.

Muffins That Are Both Moist And Easy To Consume

If muffins are moist and simple to swallow, they can be an excellent choice. Combine pureed mature bananas, almond flour, honey, eggs, and a small amount of baking powder to create banana-oat muffins. Stir-fry till golden brown. These cakes are naturally sweetened, tender, and abundant in potassium and fiber. They are an ideal choice for a short breakfast or nibble that will not cause dry mouth.

Egg Dishes Rich In Protein

Eggs are a breakfast option that is both protein-rich and versatile. Create an omelet that is packed with vegetables by combining eggs, spinach, tomatoes, bell peppers, and scallions. First, prepare the vegetables until they are tender.

Subsequently, add the whisked eggs and continue cooking until they are set. This dish supports overall health and energy levels by providing a variety of vitamins and minerals and high-quality protein from the vegetables.

Anti-Inflammatory Breakfast Ideas

To alleviate the symptoms of Sjogren's syndrome, incorporate anti-inflammatory nutrients into your breakfast. A delectable beginning can be achieved by consuming quinoa porridge that has been spiced with turmeric.

Incorporate almond milk, cinnamon, turmeric, and honey into the cooking process of quinoa. Add fresh berries and sliced almonds to the top. Turmeric possesses potent anti-inflammatory properties, while almonds and quinoa supply protein and nutritious lipids.

Sustained Energy Lunch Recipes

To sustain energy levels throughout the day, it is important to consume balanced lunches that consist of complex carbohydrates, lean proteins, and healthy lipids. For instance, consider a quinoa salad that is topped with cherry tomatoes, avocado, seared chicken, and a lemon-tahini vinaigrette. The chicken's proteins, avocado's healthy lipids, and fiber-rich quinoa contribute to the maintenance of energy and the sensation of being satisfied for an extended period.

Hearty Soups And Stews

A nutrient-dense supper that is simple to digest is best served with hearty soups and stews. A chicken and vegetable stew that includes carrots, celery, sweet potatoes, and a combination of herbs such as rosemary and thyme is a comforting example. This meal is optimal for the management of Sjogren's syndrome, as it contains a well-balanced combination of anti-inflammatory ingredients, vitamins, and proteins.

Salads That Are High In Nutrients

Compose nutrient-dense salads by incorporating a diverse array of vibrant vegetables, lean proteins, and healthy lipids. A spinach and kale salad that is topped with roasted beets, goat cheese, hazelnuts, and a balsamic vinaigrette is not only delectable but also rich in omega-3 fatty acids and antioxidants, which aid in the reduction of inflammation.

Sandwiches And Wraps That Are Simple To Prepare

Prepare wraps and sandwiches that are both nutritious and time-saving by utilizing whole grain or gluten-free wrappers that are stuffed with lean proteins and vegetables. Incorporate spinach, cucumber, and a mild mustard vinaigrette into a turkey and avocado wrap. This combination promotes overall well-being by providing essential nutrients and healthful lipids.

Anti-Inflammatory Ingredients In Grain Bowls

Grain dishes are highly adaptable and can be easily customized with anti-inflammatory ingredients. Begin by preparing a base of brown rice or quinoa. Add roasted vegetables, legumes, and a dollop of hummus on top. This meal is ideal for individuals with Sjogren's syndrome, as it provides additional anti-inflammatory advantages when sprinkled with turmeric and cumin.

Smoothies And Beverages That Are Hydrating

It is essential to maintain proper hydration, and hydrating smoothies and beverages can be both nutritious and invigorating. For an energy-boosting and hydrating beverage, combine chia seeds, banana, spinach, and coconut water in a blender. This combination aids in the management of fatigue and dehydration which are common symptoms of Sjogren's syndrome by providing electrolytes, vitamins, and omega-3s.

Dinner Recipes For Optimal Health

To achieve optimal health with Sjogren's syndrome, prioritize meals that are nutrient-dense and that mitigate inflammation. Serve a seared salmon fillet with a side of steamed broccoli and quinoa, seasoned with lemon and seasonings. This combination promotes overall well-being and reduces symptoms by providing anti-inflammatory omega-3 fatty acids from the salmon, antioxidants from the broccoli, and fiber from the quinoa.

Main Dishes That Emphasize Protein

Protein is indispensable for the preservation of immune function and muscle mass, particularly in individuals with Sjogren's syndrome. Consider baking a lean chicken breast that has been marinated in rosemary, garlic, and olive oil until it is tender. Combine this with a mixed greens salad that is garnished with avocado and a mild vinaigrette. This meal is abundant in protein and healthful lipids, which aid in tissue repair and energy levels.

Sides Of Vegetables With Lots Of Flavor

Vegetables are essential components of an anti-inflammatory diet. A mélange of colorful bell peppers, zucchini, and carrots should be roasted with a drizzle of olive oil, salt, and pepper. A delectable and nutritious side dish, roasting brings out their natural sweetness and enhances their flavors. These vegetables are a source of essential vitamins, minerals, and antioxidants that aid in the management of inflammation.

Convenient One-Pot Meals

Simplifying the preparation and cleanup process, one-pot dishes are an excellent choice for individuals with Sjogren's syndrome. Simmer lentils with minced tomatoes, spinach, carrots, and a combination of herbs and seasonings to create a satisfying lentil and vegetable stew. This dish is both nutritious and convenient, as it is abundant in plant-based protein, fiber, and essential nutrients.

Pasta And Rice Dishes That Are Low In Inflammation

Brown rice pasta combined with sautéed spinach, cherry tomatoes, and a light olive oil and garlic sauce is an option for pasta and rice dishes that promote a low-inflammatory diet. Alternatively, prepare brown rice with cumin and turmeric, and then combine it with roasted vegetables. Both options are flavorful, simple to prepare, and intended to reduce inflammation while offering a satisfying meal.

Soups And Stews That Are Hydrating

Individuals with Sjogren's syndrome require adequate hydration. Select soups and stews that are abundant in both nutrients and fluids. A classic example is a chicken and vegetable soup that is prepared with bone broth, which is rich in amino acids and collagen. Simmer the broth until all ingredients are tender, then add carrots, celery, and kale. This soup not only aids in hydration but also offers a well-balanced combination of vitamins and proteins.

<u>CHAPTER SIX</u>

Ideas For Snacks And Appetizers

Snacks That Are Both Quick And Simple To Prepare

Consider whole foods that necessitate minimal preparation for fast and effortless snacking. For instance, carrot spears with hummus, a sliced apple with peanut butter, or a sprinkling of almonds or walnuts. These foods offer a harmonious combination of fiber, healthy lipids, and protein to maintain your energy and satisfaction throughout the day.

Dips And Spreads That Are High In Nutrients

Your refreshment game can be improved by developing nutrient-dense dips and condiments. Blend avocados, chickpeas, lemon juice, garlic, and olive oil to create a homemade avocado and chickpea spread. For a nutritious and satisfying nibble, pair with whole-grain crackers or fresh vegetables such as cucumber segments, bell pepper strips, and cherry tomatoes.

Snack Bars That Reduce Inflammation

Sjogren's Syndrome symptoms are effectively managed by anti-inflammatory nutrition bars, which are effortless to prepare. Mix oats, chia seeds, flaxseeds, dried blueberries, and a small amount of honey in a mixer. Press the mixture into a baking dish, refrigerate until it is firm, and then cut it into bars. Omega-3 fatty acids and antioxidants are abundant in these bars, which aid in the mitigation of inflammation.

Fruit And Vegetable Snacks That Are Hydrating

Individuals with Sjogren's Syndrome require adequate hydration. Choose hydrating treats such as celery sticks, cucumber rounds, and watermelon segments. The high water content of these fruits and vegetables can assist in maintaining the moisture in your pharynx. Combine them with a mild dip, such as yogurt that has been combined with a small amount of honey and mint, to enhance the flavor and nutritional value.

Portable Snacks For On-The-Go

It is imperative to have portable food on hand during hectic days. Packing single-serve packets of almond butter, small packages of air-popped popcorn, or small containers of assorted nuts and dried fruits is a viable option.

These treats are convenient to transport, do not necessitate refrigeration, and offer a rapid energy boost while you are on the go.

Sweets And Snacks

Desserts That Are Nutrient-Dense And Low In Sugar

Create delectable delicacies that are both nutritious and low in sugar by incorporating natural sweeteners such as stevia, maple syrup, or honey. Incorporate ingredients that are high in nutrients, such as dark chocolate, seeds, and almonds. For instance, a chia seed pudding that is prepared with almond milk, a small amount of honey, and garnished with fresh berries provides a delectable dessert that is low in sugar.

Desserts That Are Based On Fruit That Are Hydrating

Fruit-based delicacies are an exceptional method of satisfying your sweet tooth and maintaining hydration. Consider preparing a delectable watermelon and mint salad or a fruit sorbet that incorporates blended frozen berries and a small amount of coconut water. These delicacies are not only hydrating, but they also contain essential vitamins and antioxidants.

Baked Goods That Are Anti-Inflammatory

Sjogren's Syndrome symptoms may be alleviated by baking with anti-inflammatory ingredients. Incorporate ingredients such as turmeric, ginger, and cinnamon into your recipes. For example, to enjoy a healthful and comforting delight, prepare a batch of turmeric and ginger biscuits with almond flour, honey, and a combination of these seasonings.

Dessert Recipes That Are Gluten-Free And Dairy-Free

There are numerous delectable confection alternatives available for individuals who refrain from consuming dairy and gluten. Utilize almond flour, coconut oil, and dairy-free chocolate morsels to prepare brownies that are both gluten-free and dairy-free. Another option is a coconut milk panna cotta, which is both velvety and satisfying without the presence of dairy or gluten.

Strategies For Quenching Sweet Cravings

Maintaining a supply of nutritious snacks is an effective strategy for alleviating sugary appetites. Dates, almonds, and a small amount of cocoa powder may be employed to create energy spheres.

These delights are effortless to prepare and offer a delicious dose without the use of refined sugars. For a crunchy, sweet nibble, consider roasting chickpeas with a sprinkle of cinnamon and a hint of maple syrup.

Meal Planning And Preparation

Weekly Meal Planning Strategies To facilitate meal planning for Sjogren's syndrome, develop a weekly menu that emphasizes anti-inflammatory foods. Begin by selecting meals that are high in nutrients, such as seared salmon with quinoa and steamed vegetables for dinner, oatmeal with berries for breakfast, and lentil broth for lunch. Ensure that your energy levels and nutritional requirements are met by listing the necessary ingredients and allocating a specific time each week to plan a variety of meals.

Tips for Batch Cooking and Freezing

Batch cooking can be a time- and energy-saving method. Prepare substantial quantities of chicken breasts, brown rice, and vegetable stews. For effortless reheating, divide these dishes into freezer-safe containers. For instance, prepare a substantial quantity of chili, portion it into single-serving containers, and freeze them. In this manner, you can have dishes that are ready to consume with minimal effort, thereby preserving your energy for other activities.

Grocery Shopping Guide

When conducting grocery shopping, prioritize whole foods and steer clear of processed items. Compose a list that is consistent with your dietary plan, with a focus on whole grains, lean proteins, and fresh vegetables.

Shop the perimeter of the store, which is where the fresh produce, meats, and dairy are located. If purchasing in-store is too burdensome, consider using online grocery services.

Additionally, consider enrolling in a delivery service to guarantee consistent access to fresh ingredients without overexerting yourself.

On days when energy is scarce, meals should be straightforward and rapid to prepare. Utilize kitchen appliances such as pressure cookers and slow cookers to simplify the culinary process. For example, in the morning, combine chicken, vegetables, and liquid in a slow cooker to prepare an effortless dinner. The preparation of meals can be simplified by the use of pre-chopped vegetables and pre-marinated proteins, which can reduce the amount of time required for preparation.

Adapting Family Meals For Sjogren's Syndrome

Implement minor adjustments to family meals that satisfy Sjogren's dietary requirements without the necessity of preparing separate dishes. For instance, when preparing pasta, incorporate additional vegetables and utilize whole-grain pasta.

Prepare lean proteins that are universally palatable, such as grilled chicken or fish, and accompany them with a side of anti-inflammatory vegetables. This approach ensures that the entire family consumes nutritious food while simultaneously accommodating the unique requirements of an individual with Sjogren's syndrome.

CHAPTER SEVEN

Seven-Day Meal Plan, Recipes, Ingredients, And Detailed Preparatory Guidelines For Sjogren's Syndrome

THE FIRST DAY

Breakfast: Berry Smoothie Bowl

INGREDIENTS:

• One cup of a combination of berries, including blueberries, strawberries, and raspberries

• One banana

• 1/2 cup of strained almond milk

• One tablespoon of chia seeds

• One tablespoon of almond butter

• Granola for garnishing

PREPARATION:

1. The almond milk, banana, and assorted berries should be blended until the mixture is homogeneous.

2. Transfer the mixture to a vessel and garnish with granola, almond butter, and chia seeds.

Snack: Hummus and Carrots

INGREDIENTS:

• Two large carrots, peeled and split into spears

• 1/2 cup of hummus

PREPARATION:

1. Hummus should be served with vegetable spears.

INGREDIENTS:

• One cup of prepared quinoa

• Diced cucumber, 1/2

• Diced half of a bell pepper

• Half a cup of cherry tomatoes

• 1/4 cup of finely minced herbs

• Two tablespoons of olive oil

• One teaspoonful of lemon juice

• Salt and pepper to flavor

PREPARATION:

1. Quinoa, cucumber, bell pepper, cherry tomatoes, and parsley should be combined in a sizable basin.

2. Season with salt and pepper, then drizzle with olive oil and lemon juice.

3. Combine by tossing.

INGREDIENTS:

• One apple, cut

• Two tablespoons of almond butter

PREPARATION:

1. Apple segments should be served with almond butter.

INGREDIENTS:

• One salmon tenderloin

• One tablespoon of olive oil

• Salt and pepper to flavor

• One lemon, sliced

• One broccoli head, sliced into florets

PREPARATION:

1. Turn the oven on to 375°F, or 190°C.

2. Place the salmon on a baking sheet, drizzle with olive oil, and season with salt and pepper. Add lemon segments to the top.

3. Bake the salmon for 20-25 minutes until it is fully cooked.

4. Steam broccoli for 5-7 minutes until it is tender.

5. Serve salmon with broccoli that has been steamed.

Juice: Green Detox Juice

INGREDIENTS:

• One cucumber

- Two stalks of celery

- One green apple

- Juice from half of a lemon

- One cup of spinach

- Ginger, half an inch in size

PREPARATION:

1. Blend all ingredients until they are homogeneous, and then strain them to remove the sediment.

THE SECOND DAY

Breakfast: Oatmeal with Blueberries Prepared Overnight

INGREDIENTS:

- 1/2 cup of rolled oats

- 1/2 cup of strained almond milk

• 1/4 cup of Greek yogurt

• One tablespoon of chia seeds

• One-half cup of blueberries

• Honey to be tasted

PREPARATION:

1. Combine almond milk, Greek yogurt, chia seeds, and cereals in a vessel.

2. Honey and blueberries should be incorporated.

3. Place in the refrigerator for the night.

Snack: Tzatziki with Cucumber Slices

INGREDIENTS:

• One cucumber, sliced

• 1/2 cup of tzatziki

PREPARATION:

1. Tzatziki should be served alongside cucumber segments.

Lunch: Lentil Soup

INGREDIENTS:

• One cup of drained dried legumes

• One carrot, diced

• One celery stalk, sliced

• One small onion, minced

• Two minced garlic cloves

• Four pints of vegetable broth

• One tablespoon of olive oil

• One bay leaf

• Salt and pepper to flavor

PREPARATION:

1. Heat olive oil in a sizable kettle over medium heat. Add the carrot, celery, and onion, and sauté until they are tender.

2. Add garlic and simmer for one minute.

3. Combine lentils, vegetable broth, and bay leaf. Bring the mixture to a boil, then reduce the heat and allow it to simmer for 30 to 40 minutes until the lentils are soft.

4. Add salt and pepper to taste.

Snack: Almonds

INGREDIENTS:

• 1/4 cup of pistachios

PREPARATION:

1. Serve hazelnuts as a refreshment.

INGREDIENTS:

• One chicken breast

• One tablespoon of olive oil

• Salt and pepper to flavor

• One cup of prepared quinoa

• One bundle of asparagus, trimmed

• Juice from one lemon

PREPARATION:

1. Preheat the grill to medium-high fire.

2. Season chicken breast with salt, pepper, and olive oil.

3. Grill poultry for 6-7 minutes on each side until it is thoroughly cooked.

4. Steam asparagus for 4-5 minutes until it is tender.

5. Grilled chicken is served with asparagus and quinoa, which are drizzled with lemon juice.

Carrot-orange juice:

INGREDIENTS:

• Three vegetables

• Two oranges, peeled

• Ginger, half an inch in size

PREPARATION:

1. Blend all ingredients until they are homogeneous, and then strain them to remove the sediment.

THIRD DAY

INGREDIENTS:

• One piece of whole-grain bread

• Mashed half of an avocado

• One egg

• Salt and pepper to flavor

• Red pepper sprinkles (optional)

PREPARATION:

1. Toast the bread.

2. Spread pureed avocado on toast and season with salt and pepper.

3. Place the egg on top of the avocado toast after it has been poached. If preferred, garnish with red pepper granules.

INGREDIENTS:

• Two celery stalks, split into pieces

• Two tablespoons of peanut butter

PREPARATION:

1. Peanut butter should be served with celery stalks.

INGREDIENTS:

• Two cups of fresh spinach

• One cup of cut strawberries

• 1/4 cup of shredded feta cheese

• 1/4 cup of sliced almonds

• Two tablespoons of balsamic vinaigrette

PREPARATION:

1. Spinach, strawberries, feta cheese, and pistachios should be combined in a sizable bowl.

2. Drizzle the balsamic vinaigrette over the salad and toss to incorporate.

Snack: A Variety of Berries

INGREDIENTS:

• One cup of a combination of berries, including blueberries, strawberries, and raspberries

PREPARATION:

1. As a refreshment, serve a variety of fruit.

Dinner: Stuffed Bell Peppers

INGREDIENTS:

• Two bell peppers, seeded and divided

• One cup of brown rice that has been prepared

• 1/2 cup of black beans, rinsed and drained

• 1/2 cup of maize kernels

• 1/2 cup of diced tomatoes

• 1/4 cup of grated cheese (optional)

• One teaspoon of cumin

• Salt and pepper to flavor

PREPARATION:

1. Preheat the oven to 375°F (190°C).

2. Brown rice, black beans, maize, diced tomatoes, cumin, salt, and pepper should be combined in a basin.

3. Fill the bell peppers with the rice mixture and set them in a roasting dish.

4. If desirable, garnish with grated cheese.

5. Bake the peppers for 25-30 minutes until they are soft.

Apple and beetroot juice

INGREDIENTS:

• One beetroot, skinned and sliced

• Two apples, trimmed and sliced

• Juice from half of a lemon

PREPARATION:

1. Blend all ingredients until they are homogeneous, and then strain them to remove the sediment.

THE FOURTH DAY

Breakfast: Mango Chia Pudding

INGREDIENTS:

• 1/4 cup of chia seeds

• One cup of strained almond milk

• One tablespoon of honey

• Diced mango, 1/2

PREPARATION:

1. Chia seeds, almond milk, and honey should be combined in a basin. Mix thoroughly.

2. Place in the refrigerator for a minimum of four hours or overnight.

3. Before serving, garnish with diced mango.

Snack: Guacamole with Sliced Bell Peppers

INGREDIENTS:

• One sliced bell pepper

• 1/2 cup of guacamole

PREPARATION:

1. Guacamole should be served alongside bell pepper segments.

Mediterranean Chickpea Salad for Lunch

INGREDIENTS:

• One can of legumes, rinsed and drained

• Diced cucumber, 1/2

• Diced half of a bell pepper

• Diced 1/4 cup of red scallion

• Sliced kalamata olives, 1/4 cup

• Crumbled 1/4 cup of feta cheese

• Two tablespoons of olive oil

• One teaspoonful of lemon juice

• Salt and pepper to flavor

PREPARATION:

1. Chickpeas, cucumber, bell pepper, red onion, olives, and feta cheese should be combined in a sizable basin.

2. Season with salt and pepper, then drizzle with olive oil and lemon juice.

3. Combine by tossing.

Snack: Edamame

INGREDIENTS:

• One cup of steamed edamame, drizzled with sea salt

PREPARATION:

1. Sprinkle sea salt over steamed edamame before serving.

INGREDIENTS:

- One pound of minced turkey

- 1/4 cup of almond flour

- One egg

- 1/4 cup of grated Parmesan cheese

- One minced garlic clove

- One teaspoon of dried oregano

- Salt and pepper to flavor

- Two spiralized zucchinis

- One cup of marinara sauce

PREPARATION:

1. Preheat the oven to 375°F (190°C).

2. Combine minced turkey, almond flour, egg, Parmesan cheese, garlic, oregano, salt, and pepper in a basin. Combine thoroughly.

3. Shape the mixture into meatballs and arrange them on a baking sheet.

4. Bake for 20-25 minutes until the food is fully finished.

5. Sauté zucchini noodles in a pan over medium heat until they are tender, while the meatballs are roasting.

6. Serve the meatballs over zucchini linguine and drizzle with marinara sauce.

INGREDIENTS:

• One half of a pineapple, trimmed and sliced

• One cucumber, sliced

• Juice from half of a lime

PREPARATION:

1.   Blend all ingredients until they are homogeneous, and then strain them to remove the sediment.

DAY FIVE

Breakfast: Nuts and Greek Yogurt with Honey

INGREDIENTS:

• One cup of Greek yogurt

• One tablespoon of honey

• 1/4 cup of a combination of nuts, including pistachios, walnuts, and almonds

PREPARATION:

1. Serve Greek yogurt with honey and a variety of almonds.

Snack: Walnuts and Sliced Pear

INGREDIENTS:

• One cut pear

• 1/4 cup of walnuts

PREPARATION:

1. Walnuts should be served alongside pear segments.

Lunch: Turkey and Avocado Wrap

INGREDIENTS:

• One whole-grain tortilla

• Three slices of turkey breast

• One half of an avocado, divided

• 1/4 cup of assorted greens

• One teaspoonful of hummus

PREPARATION:

1. Apply hummus to the tortilla.

2. Arrange turkey, avocado, and assorted greens in a layer.

3. Fold the tortilla in half and roll it up.

Snack: Mozzarella with Cherry Tomatoes

INGREDIENTS:

• One cup of cherry tomatoes

• 1/4 cup of mozzarella patties

• One teaspoonful of balsamic vinegar

PREPARATION:

1. Combine mozzarella patties and cherry tomatoes with balsamic vinegar.

Dinner: Grilled Shrimp with Quinoa and Asparagus

INGREDIENTS:

• Peeled and deveined shrimp, weighing half a pound

• One tablespoon of olive oil

• One teaspoon of garlic powder

• Salt and pepper to flavor

• One cup of prepared quinoa

• One bundle of asparagus, trimmed

• Juice from one lemon

PREPARATION:

1. Preheat the grill to medium-high fire.

2. Combine shellfish with garlic powder, olive oil, salt, and pepper.

3. Grill shrimp for 2-3 minutes on each side until they are fully cooked.

4. Steam asparagus for 4-5 minutes until it is tender.

5. Grilled prawns should be served with asparagus and quinoa, finished with a drizzle of lemon juice.

Juice: Mint-Watermelon Juice

INGREDIENTS:

• Two cups of sliced melons

• One-half cup of fresh mint leaves

• Juice from half of a lime

PREPARATION:

1. Blend all ingredients until they are homogeneous, and then strain them to remove the sediment.

SIXTH DAY

Breakfast: Spinach and banana smoothie

INGREDIENTS:

• One banana

• One cup of spinach

• 1/2 cup of strained almond milk

• One tablespoon of almond butter

• One tablespoon of flaxseeds

PREPARATION:

1. All ingredients should be blended until they are homogeneous.

INGREDIENTS:

• One sliced red bell pepper

• 1/2 cup of hummus

PREPARATION:

1. Hummus should be served with red bell pepper segments.

INGREDIENTS:

• 1/2 cup of kidney beans, strained and rinsed

• 1/2 cup of legumes, rinsed and drained

• 1/2 cup of black beans, rinsed and drained

• 1/4 cup of diced red scallion

• 1/4 cup of minced cilantro

• Two tablespoons of olive oil

• One tablespoon of red wine vinegar

• Salt and pepper to flavor

PREPARATION:

1. Kidney beans, lentils, black beans, red onion, and cilantro should be combined in a sizable receptacle.

2. Season with salt and pepper, then drizzle with red wine vinegar and olive oil.

3. Combine by tossing.

Snack: Pineapple Chunks

INGREDIENTS:

• One cup of pineapple slices

PREPARATION:

1. As a refreshment, offer pineapple pieces.

INGREDIENTS:

• One cod fillet

• One tablespoon of olive oil

• Salt and pepper to flavor

• One sweet potato, trimmed and cubed

• One cup of trimmed green beans

PREPARATION:

1. Preheat the oven to 375°F (190°C).

2. Place the cod on a baking sheet, drizzle with olive oil, and season with salt and pepper.

3. Place green asparagus and sweet potato cubes around the cod.

4. Bake for 20-25 minutes until the cod is fully cooked and the vegetables are tender.

INGREDIENTS:

• Two oranges, peeled

• Ginger, half an inch in size

PREPARATION:

1. Blend all ingredients until they are homogeneous, and then strain them to remove the sediment.

SEVENTH DAY

Breakfast: Buckwheat pancakes with berries

INGREDIENTS:

• 1/2 cup of buckwheat flour

• 1/2 cup of strained almond milk

* One egg

* 1 tablespoon of heated coconut oil

* 1/2 teaspoon of baking powder

* 1/2 cup of various fruit

* Maple syrup for drizzling

PREPARATION:

1. Buckwheat flour, almond milk, egg, coconut oil, and baking powder are combined in a basin.

2. Preheat a non-stick skillet over medium heat and pour in the batter to create crepes.

3. Cook until bubbles appear on the surface, then rotate and continue cooking until the surface is golden brown.

4. Serve with a drizzle of maple syrup and a variety of fruit.

INGREDIENTS:

• One mango, skinned and cut

PREPARATION:

1. Mango segments may be served as refreshment.

Lunch: Chickpea and Avocado Salad

INGREDIENTS:

• One can of legumes, rinsed and drained

• One avocado, minced

• Diced cucumber, 1/2

• Diced 1/4 cup of red scallion

• Two tablespoons of olive oil

• One teaspoonful of lemon juice

• Salt and pepper to flavor

PREPARATION:

1. Chickpeas, avocado, cucumber, and red onion should be combined in a sizable basin.

2. Season with salt and pepper, then drizzle with olive oil and lemon juice.

3. Combine by tossing.

Snack: Trail Mix

INGREDIENTS:

• 1/4 cup of pistachios

• 1/4 cup of dried cranberries

• 1/4 cup of pumpkin seeds

PREPARATION:

1. Combine all ingredients and serve as a refreshment.

INGREDIENTS:

• One split poultry breast

• One tablespoon of olive oil

• One sliced red bell pepper

• One sliced yellow bell pepper

• One cup of broccoli florets

• One sliced carrot

• Two teaspoons of low-sodium soy sauce

• One teaspoon of sesame oil

• One minced garlic clove

• One teaspoon of minced ginger

PREPARATION:

1. In a sizable skillet, heat olive oil over medium-high heat.

2. Add chicken slices and sauté until they are fully cooked and caramelized. Remove from the skillet and place it aside.

3. Bell peppers, broccoli, and carrots should be incorporated into the same skillet. Continue cooking until the vegetables are golden and tender.

4. Return the poultry to the skillet. Combine garlic, ginger, sesame oil, and soy sauce.

5. Combine by tossing and continue cooking for an additional 2-3 minutes.

INGREDIENTS:

• One-half cup of strawberries

• One-half cup of blueberries

• 1/2 cup of raspberries

• One-half of an apple, skinned and sliced

PREPARATION:

1. Blend all ingredients until they are homogeneous, and then strain them to remove the sediment.

CHAPTER EIGHT

Seven Desserts Procedural Recipes For Sjogren's Syndrome And Guidelines

1. Hydration: Choose foods that are high in water content to alleviate parched mouth and eyes.

2. Anti-inflammatory: Incorporate ingredients that are abundant in omega-3 fatty acids, antioxidants, and other anti-inflammatory properties.

3. Comfortable to Consume: Soft textures are indispensable for alleviating discomfort during meals.

4. Sugar Management: Reduce the consumption of added sugars to prevent excessive blood sugar levels, which can exacerbate symptoms.

5. Nutrient-Dense: Emphasize nutrient-dense diets to promote immune system health and maintain overall health.

INGREDIENTS:

• One cup of almond milk

• Three tablespoons of chia seeds

• One cup of assorted berries, either fresh or frozen

• One tablespoon of maple syrup or honey

• One teaspoon of vanilla extract

STEPS:

1. In a basin, combine almond milk, chia seeds, honey, and vanilla extract.

2. Stir the mixture thoroughly to ensure that the chia seeds are evenly distributed.

3. The mixture should be refrigerated for a minimum of four hours or overnight until it reaches a pudding-like consistency.

4. Before serving, garnish with a variety of berries.

2. CHOCOLATE AVOCADO MOUSSE

INGREDIENTS:

• Two mature avocados

• 1/4 cup of cocoa powder

• 1/4 cup of maple syrup or honey

• One teaspoon of vanilla extract

• A mere sprinkle of salt

STEPS:

1. In a food processor, combine all ingredients until they are uniformly blended.

2. Evaluate the sweetness and make any necessary adjustments.

3. Place in the refrigerator for a minimum of one hour before serving.

3. BANANA NICE CREAM

INGREDIENTS:

• Three fully mature avocados

• 1/2 teaspoon of vanilla extract

• Nuts, berries, or desiccated coconut are optional garnishes.

STEPS:

1. Slice bananas and chill them for a minimum of two hours.

2. Blend vanilla extract and frozen banana slices until they are smooth and creamy.

3. Garnish with optional garnishes and serve immediately.

4. ALMONDS AND HONEY IN COCONUT YOGURT

INGREDIENTS:

• One cup of coconut yogurt

• One tablespoon of honey

• 1/4 cup of slivered almonds

STEPS:

1. Spoon coconut yogurt into a dish.

2. Apply honey to the yogurt.

3. Sprinkle with slivered almonds.

4. Chill before serving.

INGREDIENTS:

• Four apples

• 1/4 cup of raisins

• 1/4 cup of chopped walnuts

• One tablespoon of honey

• One teaspoon of cinnamon

STEPS:

1. Set the oven's temperature to 175°C/350°F.

2. Core the apples, ensuring that the bottom remains unaffected.

3. Combine raisins, walnuts, honey, and cinnamon in a small basin.

4. Fill each apple with the mixture.

5. Arrange the apples in a baking dish that contains a small amount of water at the bottom.

6. Bake the fruits for 25-30 minutes until they are soft.

6. MANGO SMOOTHIE

INGREDIENTS:

• One succulent mango

• One-half cup of Greek yogurt

• 1/2 cup of coconut water

• One tablespoon of honey

• A small quantity of ice crystals

STEPS:

1. Chop the mango and peel it.

2. Blend mango, Greek yogurt, coconut water, honey, and ice crystals until the mixture is homogeneous.

3. Serve immediately.

7. OATMEAL COOKIES

INGREDIENTS:

• One cup of rolled oats

• One-half cup of almond flour

• 1/2 teaspoon of baking soda

• 1/4 cup of honey

• 1/4 cup of heated coconut oil

• One teaspoon of vanilla extract

• 1/2 cup of raisins

STEPS:

1. Preheat the oven to 350°F (175°C).

2. Combine almond flour, baking soda, and cereals in a basin.

3. Combine the dry ingredients with honey, liquefied coconut oil, and vanilla extract. Combine thoroughly.

4. Incorporate the raisins by folding them in.

5. Place tiny quantities of the mixture onto a baking sheet that has been lined with parchment paper.

6. Bake for 10-12 minutes until the surface is a rich golden color.

In conclusion, mindful dietary practices, which prioritize hydration, anti-inflammatory ingredients, and easily digestible textures, are essential for adhering to a diet that is appropriate for Sjogren's Syndrome. These seven confection recipes offer a diverse array of flavors and textures that are both delectable and suitable for those with dietary restrictions.

Individuals with Sjogren's Syndrome can more effectively manage their symptoms and experience a balanced, fulfilling diet by concentrating on these guidelines.

CHAPTER NINE

Seven Smoothie Procedural Recipes For Sjogren's Syndrome And Guidelines

The primary symptoms of Sjogren's Syndrome are parched mouth and dry eyes, which are the result of an autoimmune disorder that affects the organs that produce moisture.

It is essential to maintain hydration and consume a diet that is well-balanced and contains anti-inflammatory foods to effectively manage these symptoms. Smoothies can be an exceptional complement to the diet of an individual with Sjogren's Syndrome. They are simple to consume, hydrating, and can be rich in nutrients that promote overall health and inflammation reduction. The following are seven smoothie recipes that are explicitly intended to be beneficial for individuals with Sjogren's Syndrome, as well as instructions for preparing your nutrient-rich smoothies.

Smoothie Recipe Guidelines

1. Hydration: Consume fruits and vegetables that are high in water content, such as melons, watermelon, and berries.

2. Healthy Fats: To facilitate nutrient assimilation, incorporate sources of healthy fats such as avocado, chia seeds, and flaxseeds.

3. Anti-Inflammatory Ingredients: Incorporate ingredients such as turmeric, ginger, and leafy greens to mitigate inflammation.

4. Protein: Incorporate protein sources such as Greek yogurt, almond butter, or protein powder to help maintain muscle mass and keep you fuller for longer.

5. Natural Sweeteners: If necessary, utilize natural sweeteners such as honey or dates; however, prioritize the natural sweetness of fruits.

6. Variation: To prevent monotony and guarantee a diverse array of nutrients, it is important to rotate ingredients.

1. GREEN SMOOTHIE WITH HYDRATION

INGREDIENTS:

• One cup of spinach

• One-half of a cucumber, trimmed and sliced

• One green apple, cored and sliced

• One-skinned kiwi

• One-half of an avocado

• One tablespoon of chia seeds

• One cup of coconut water

STEPS:

1. Add the avocado, kiwi, green apple, spinach, and cucumber to a blender.

2. The chia seeds should be sprinkled in.

3. Pour the coconut water into the container.

4. Blend until the mixture is velvety and smooth.

5. For a hydrating and revitalizing beverage, serve immediately.

2. BERRY ANTIOXIDANT SMOOTHIE

INGREDIENTS:

• One cup of a combination of berries, including raspberries, blueberries, and strawberries

• One-half of a banana

• One tablespoon of ground flaxseeds

• One-half cup of Greek yogurt

• One cup of almond milk

STEPS:

1. Combine the almond milk, Greek yogurt, pulverized flaxseeds, banana, and assorted berries in a blender.

2. Blend until the mixture is uniform.

3. Pour into a glass and relish a smoothie that is antioxidant-rich and nutrient-dense.

3. TROPICAL TURMERIC SMOOTHIE

INGREDIENTS:

• One cup of pineapple slices

• One-half mango, trimmed and sliced

• 1/2 teaspoon of turmeric powder

• 1/4 teaspoon of ginger powder

• One tablespoon of coconut oil

• One cup of citrus juice

STEPS:

1. Combine the coconut oil, turmeric powder, ginger powder, pineapple, and mango in a Vitamix.

2. Incorporate the citrus juice.

3. Blend until the mixture is velvety and smooth.

4. Indulge in the anti-inflammatory properties and tropical flavors.

4. SMOOTHIE WITH AVOCADO AND BERRIES

INGREDIENTS:

• One-half of an avocado

• One-half cup of blueberries

• One-half cup of strawberries

• One tablespoon of hemp seeds

• One cup of unadulterated coconut milk

STEPS:

1. Combine the avocado, blueberries, strawberries, and hemp seeds in a Vitamix.

2. Pour the coconut milk into the container.

3. Blend until the mixture is viscous and smooth.

4. For a nutritious, creamy beverage, serve promptly.

5. ENERGY-BOOSTING MATCHA SMOOTHIE

INGREDIENTS:

• One teaspoon of matcha powder

• One-half of a banana

• One cup of spinach

• One tablespoon of almond butter

• One cup of oat milk

STEPS:

1. In a blender, combine the banana, spinach, almond butter, oat milk, and matcha powder.

2. Blend until the mixture is well-integrated and homogeneous.

3. Experience an increase in vitality and antioxidants.

6. CITRUS SUNSHINE SMOOTHIE

INGREDIENTS:

• One orange, skinned and segmented

• One-half grapefruit, peeled and segmented

• One-half cup of carrot juice

• One tablespoon of chia seeds

• One cup of water

STEPS:

1. Combine the citrus, grapefruit, carrot juice, and chia seeds in a blender.

2. Add the water.

3. Blend until the mixture is uniform.

4. Take pleasure in the vitamin C boost and the vibrant, citrus flavors.

7. BANANA OAT SMOOTHIE WITH NUTS

INGREDIENTS:

• One banana

• 1/4 cup of toasted oats

• One tablespoon of peanut butter

• One tablespoon of honey

• One cup of strained almond milk

STEPS:

1. Mix the peanut butter, honey, banana, and rolled oats in a Vitamix.

2. Incorporate the almond milk.

3. Blend until the mixture is velvety and smooth.

4. For a nutritious and satisfying smoothie, serve immediately.

In summary, these cocktails are intended to alleviate inflammation, promote hydration, and supply essential nutrients to individuals who are coping with Sjogren's Syndrome.

Please feel at liberty to experiment with the ingredients and modify the recipes to accommodate your dietary requirements and personal preferences. Consume these nutritious and delightful smoothies as an integral component of your well-rounded diet.

CHAPTER TEN

Lifestyle Suggestions For The Management Of Sjogren's Syndrome

Ensured Hydration Throughout the Day: Individuals with Sjogren's Syndrome need to maintain sufficient hydration levels to alleviate symptoms such as parched mouth and dry eyes. This entails consuming hydrating foods, such as fruits and vegetables, and consuming an abundance of water throughout the day.

Using a water vessel with measurements can assist in monitoring daily intake, to consume a minimum of 8 glasses (64 ounces) of water each day. Additionally, eliminating beverages that dehydrate the body, such as caffeine and alcohol, can bolster hydration efforts.

It is crucial to integrate stress-management strategies into one's daily routine, as tension can exacerbate the symptoms of Sjogren's Syndrome. Meditation, yoga, and deep breathing exercises can all contribute to the reduction of tension levels. Setting boundaries, prioritizing duties, and establishing a tranquil environment at home are also effective strategies for preventing overwhelm. Effective stress management can be achieved by maintaining a journal to monitor stress triggers and implementing coping mechanisms as necessary.

Regular exercise is advantageous for individuals with Sjogren's Syndrome, as it enhances their general health and alleviates symptoms such as fatigue and joint discomfort. Walking, swimming, and yoga are low-impact exercises that offer substantial health benefits while being mild on the joints. Strive to engage in moderate exercise for a minimum of 30 minutes on most days of the week, progressively increasing the intensity and duration as tolerated.

Consulting with a physical therapist or healthcare provider can assist in the customization of an exercise regimen to meet the unique requirements and constraints of each individual.

Tips For Improved Rest And Recovery

Quality sleep is crucial for the management of Sjogren's Syndrome symptoms and the promotion of overall well-being. Ensuring a consistent sleep schedule, optimizing the sleep environment, and establishing a relaxing twilight regimen are essential components of enhancing sleep quality. Better sleep can be achieved by avoiding stimulating activities and electronic devices before bedtime, ensuring a comfortable mattress and pillows, and maintaining a cold and dark bedroom. If sleep disturbances persist, it may be necessary to consult with a healthcare provider regarding potential solutions, such as sleep therapy or medications.

Community Support And Resources

Valuable support and resources can be obtained by establishing connections with others who comprehend the difficulties associated with living with Sjogren's Syndrome.

Individuals can exchange advice, share experiences, and access pertinent information by participating in online forums, support groups, or social media communities that are specifically dedicated to Sjogren's Syndrome. Furthermore, locating reputable websites, publications, and organizations that specialize in Sjogren's

Syndrome can offer a wealth of educational materials, comprehensive resources, and the most recent information on research and treatment options. Engaging with the Sjogren's Syndrome community can cultivate a sense of empowerment and belonging that is essential for the effective management of the condition.

Conclusion

The significance of customized nutritional strategies to alleviate symptoms and enhance the quality of life for individuals afflicted with this autoimmune disorder is emphasized by the conclusion regarding a Sjögren's syndrome diet.

Sjögren's syndrome does not have a universally prescribed diet; however, an anti-inflammatory diet that is abundant in fruits, vegetables, whole cereals, and lean proteins can be beneficial in reducing systemic inflammation.

Omega-3 fatty acids, which are abundant in flaxseed and fish, are notably advantageous due to their anti-inflammatory properties.

It is imperative to increase fluid intake and incorporate hydrating foods, as Sjögren's syndrome frequently induces dehydration, necessitating the importance of hydration. Symptoms can be alleviated by avoiding trigger foods, including those that are high in sugar, caffeine, and artificial preservatives. Furthermore, it may be advantageous for patients to refrain from consuming gluten and dairy, as these substances may exacerbate inflammation in certain individuals.

Gut health, which is increasingly acknowledged to be associated with autoimmune conditions, can be bolstered by probiotics and fermented foods.

A personalized approach, which is frequently devised in consultation with healthcare providers and nutritionists, is advised due to the potential for individual responses to dietary changes to vary.

In general, diet is essential for the management of symptoms and the improvement of overall well-being, even though it is unable to cure Sjögren's syndrome.

THE END

www.ingramcontent.com/pod-product-compliance
Lightning Source LLC
Chambersburg PA
CBHW061049250726
48653CB00001B/318